As You Grow

A MODERN MEMORY BOOK FOR BABY

Korie Herold

paige tate
& CO.

paige tate
& CO.

Published in 2018 by Blue Star Press
Paige Tate & Co. is an imprint of Blue Star Press
PO Box 5622, Bend, OR 97708
contact@paigetate.com | www.paigetate.com

Illustrations and Design by Korie Herold

ISBN: 9781944515478
Printed in China

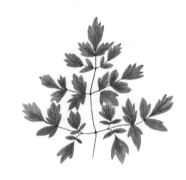

Baby, it's a long story. You better
snuggle up and get comfortable.

Love, Mama

Each and every page of this book was delicately crafted, illustrated, and painted by hand, by a single artist
located in Kingwood, TX. Learn more about the artist behind this book in the pages following the journal section.

What's Inside

HELPFUL TIPS TO GET THE MOST OUT OF YOUR BOOK

I created this book with a desire for a baby book that is gender neutral in its design, elegant in its simplicity, and a joy to record precious memories in. My hope is that this will become a cherished book to one day gift to your baby.

As You Grow can be customized to reflect your unique and wonderful family. This book allows you to celebrate your particular family dynamics, and the holidays and seasons that your family enjoys together. The spiral binding allows you to easily remove any pages you wish to. For example, if you can't remember a lick of your pregnancy, you can even remove this entire section so you are not faced with empty pages you'll never fill out! The recommended method to remove pages is with the careful use of scissors, rather than tearing pages out by hand.

To get the most out of your book, each section has pockets to hold cherished memories from that time: cards to baby, notes from grandparents, first artwork, special photographs, and so forth.

For quality and consistency, I recommend that you use a black archival ink pen within the pages. I use Micron® pens.

I would love to see how you are making your copy of As You Grow your own on social media! Let's use the hashtag #asyougrowBOOK to stay connected.

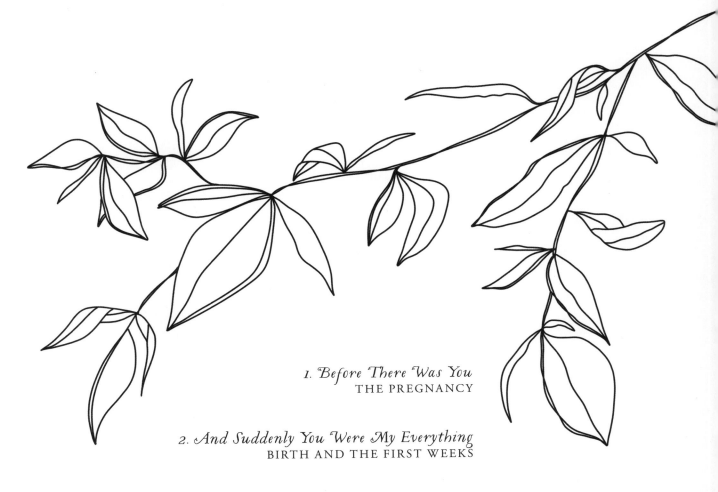

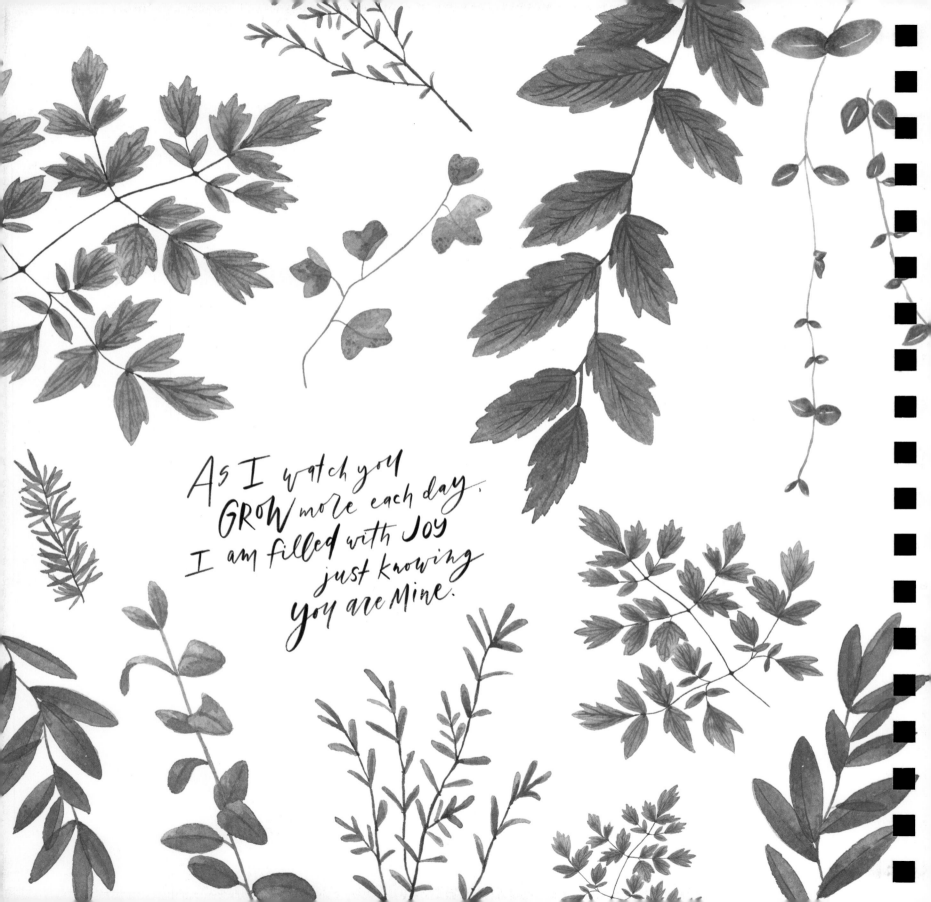

As I watch you
GROW more each day,
I am filled with JOY
just knowing
you are mine.

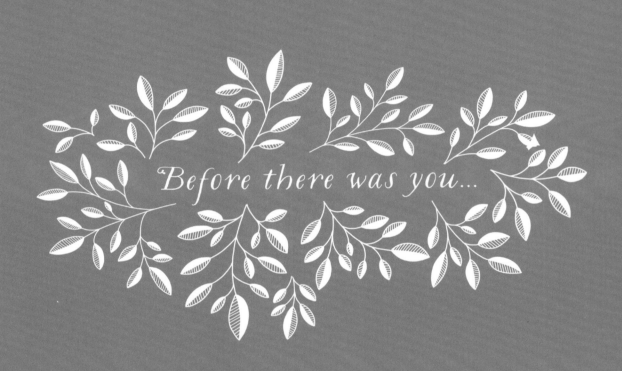

Before there was you...

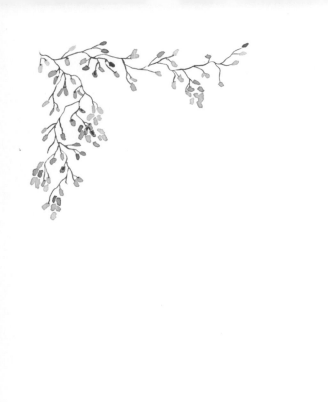
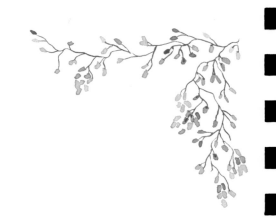
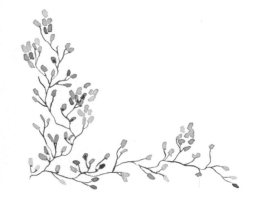
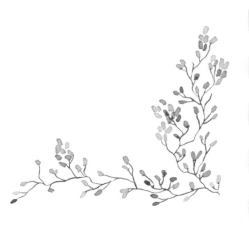

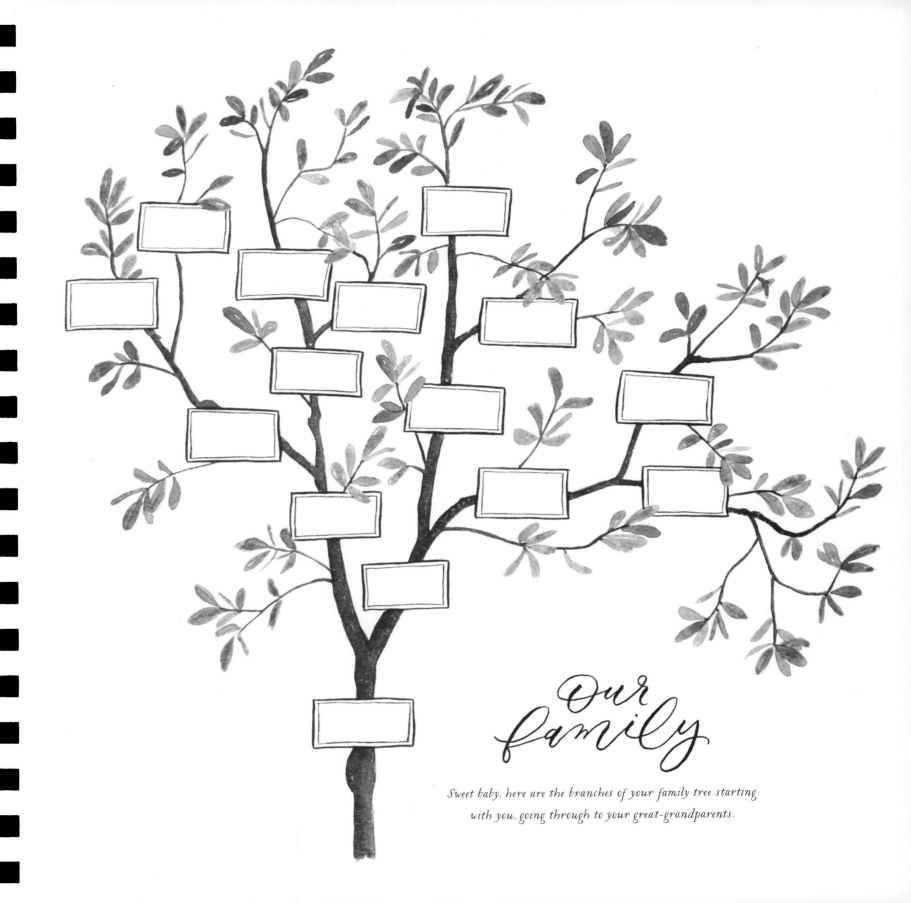

Our family

Sweet baby, here are the branches of your family tree starting
with you, going through to your great-grandparents.

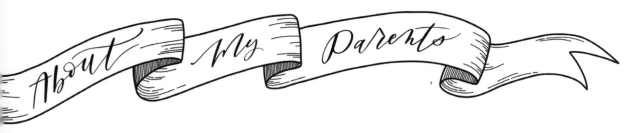

About My Parents

What I hope you will call me: _____

_____

My full name: _____

_____

Birthday: _____

_____

Born in: _____

_____

Grew up in: _____

_____

My best friends: _____

_____

Traits you got from me: _____

_____

A memory from my childhood I want to share with you: _____

_____

_____

_____

_____

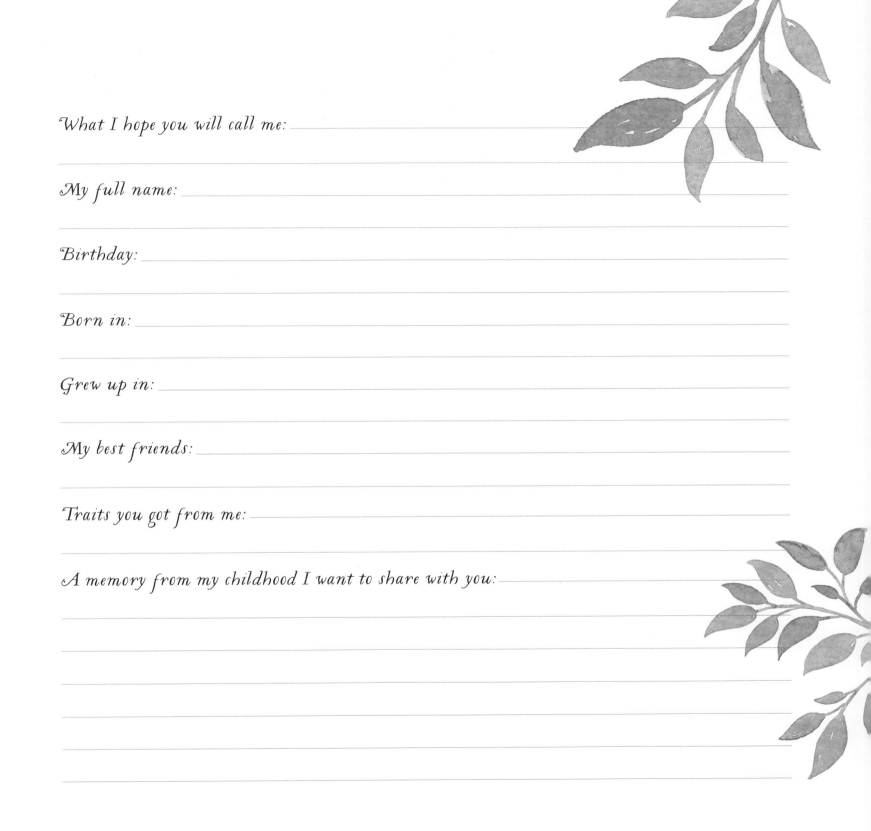

What I hope you will call me: _____

_____

My full name: _____

_____

Birthday: _____

_____

Born in: _____

_____

Grew up in: _____

_____

My best friends: _____

_____

Traits you got from me: _____

_____

A memory from my childhood I want to share with you: _____

_____

_____

_____

_____

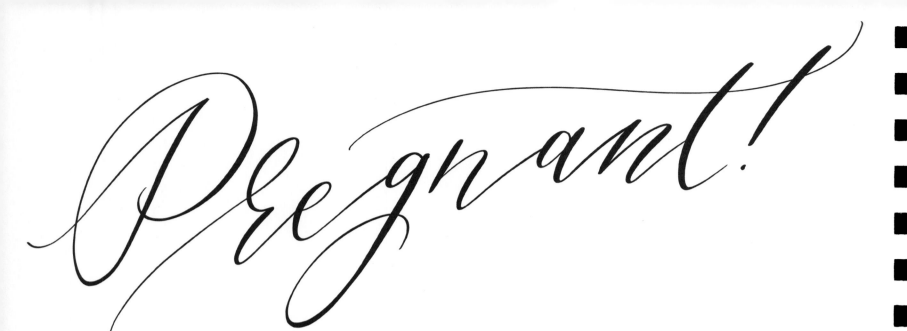

Pregnant!

Date I found out about you: _____

_____

My reaction to finding out: _____

_____

_____

_____

_____

_____

_____

_____

_____

_____

_____

_____

How friends & family heard the news: _____

_____

_____

_____

Who had the best reaction? _____

_____

Date I first heard your heartbeat: _____

_____

Date of first ultrasound: _____

_____

Date I felt first kick: _____

_____

Date someone else felt a kick: Who? _____

_____

Before you were born I called you: _____

_____

Nervous about: _____

_____

Three words to describe this pregnancy: _____

_____

Food I craved while pregnant: _____

_____

Food aversions and things that made me sick: _____

_____

Add Photo Here!

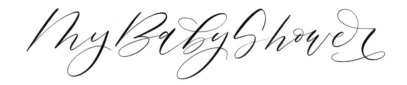

My Baby Shower

Date: _____

_____

Place shower was held: _____

_____

Hosted by: _____

_____

Who attended: _____

_____

_____

_____

How many people rubbed my belly: _____

_____

What I wore: _____

_____

What we did at the shower: _____

_____

_____

_____

Add Photo Here!

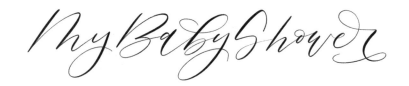

My Baby Shower

Date: _____

_____

Place shower was held: _____

_____

Hosted by: _____

_____

Who attended: _____

_____

_____

_____

How many people rubbed my belly: _____

_____

What I wore: _____

_____

What we did at the shower: _____

_____

_____

_____

_____

Thoughts before your big arrival:

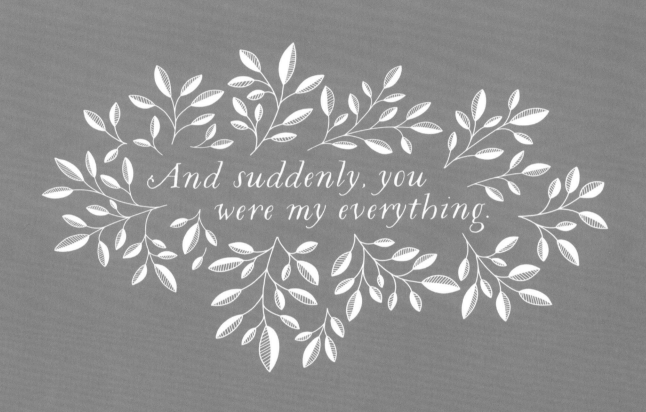

And suddenly, you were my everything.

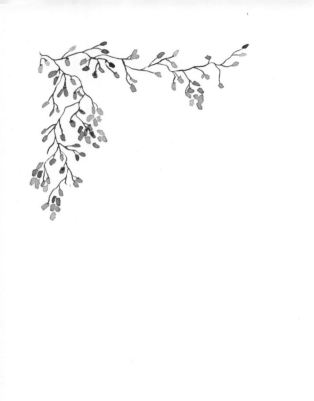
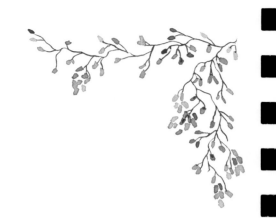
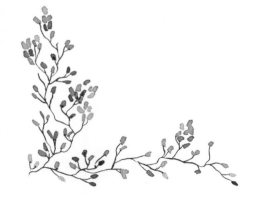
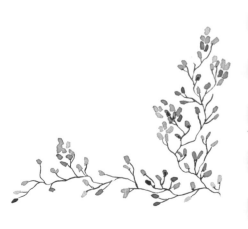

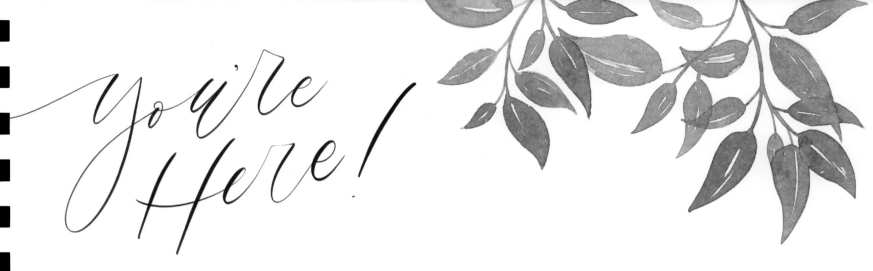

You're Here!

Date: _____

_____

Your height & weight: _____

_____

Time of birth: _____

_____

Where: _____

_____

Feelings: _____

_____

The weather was like this the day you were born: _____

_____

_____

How your name was chosen: _____

_____

_____

_____

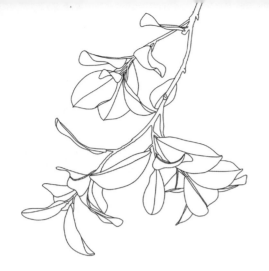

Add Birth Photo Here!

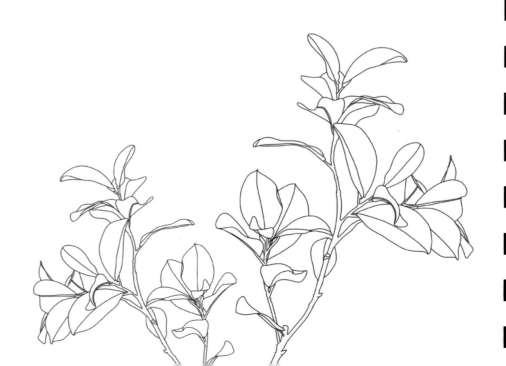

Baby's First Little Footprints

Birth Story

Consider having the birth story told by more than one person.
Did anyone besides Mom experience the birth?

Birth Story

Birth Story

Add Photo Here!

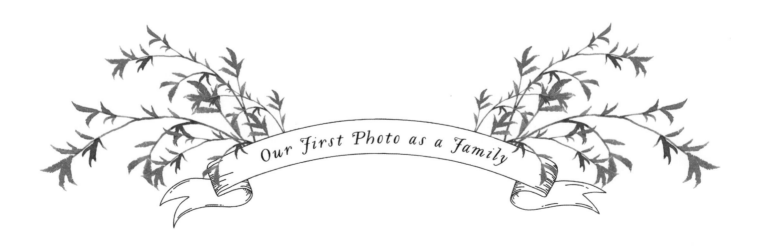

Our First Photo as a Family

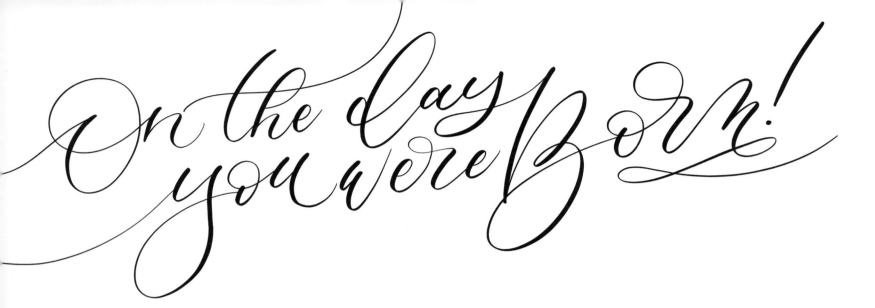

On the day you were Born!

Our government leader: _____

_____

Major news or headlines today: _____

_____

_____

_____

#1 Movie (and last movie we saw in theaters): _____

_____

#1 Billboard song (and Mom's current favorite song): _____

_____

Best TV show currently airing (and current binge show): ___

_____

_____

_____

Famous people who share a birthday with you: _____

_____

Fashion trends: _____

_____

_____

_____

Average prices:

Milk: _____

_____

Soda: _____

_____

Gas: _____

_____

Newspaper: _____

_____

Postage: _____

_____

Movie Ticket: _____

_____

Special First Days

Who changed the first diaper, and what was their skill level? How did it go?

_____

_____

_____

Visitors during the first 48 hours:

Who?	Miles Traveled	Duration of Stay	First Reaction to You

Use this page however you see fit. For example, if you want to tell another story from the birthing experience, here is your chance!

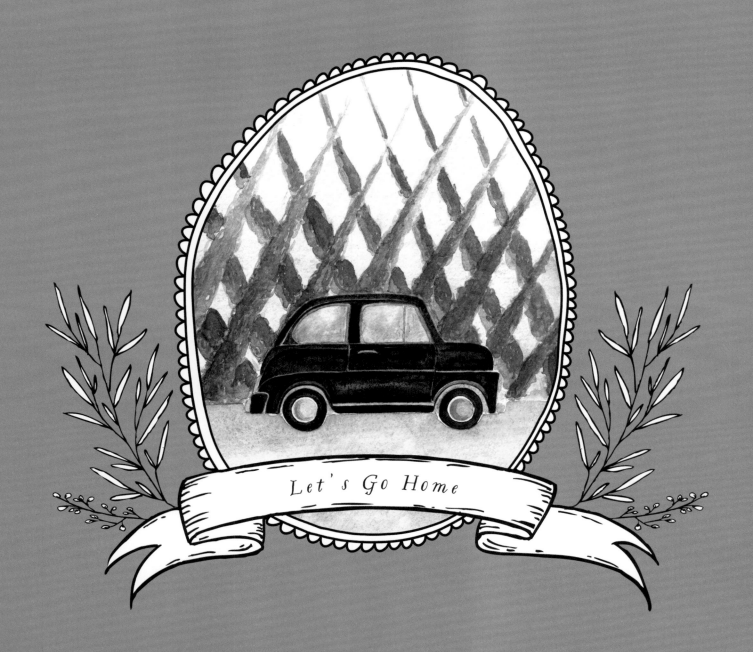

Let's Go Home

With you, I am Home.

Address: _____

_____

Pets: _____

_____

Siblings: _____

_____

Your first outfit: _____

_____

_____

Photo of our home

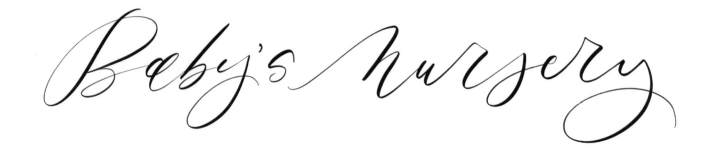

Baby's Nursery

Theme/color palette/special touches: _____

_____

_____

_____

How the room makes me feel: _____

_____

_____

_____

What I thought about as I got your nursery ready: _____

_____

_____

_____

_____

_____

_____

_____

_____

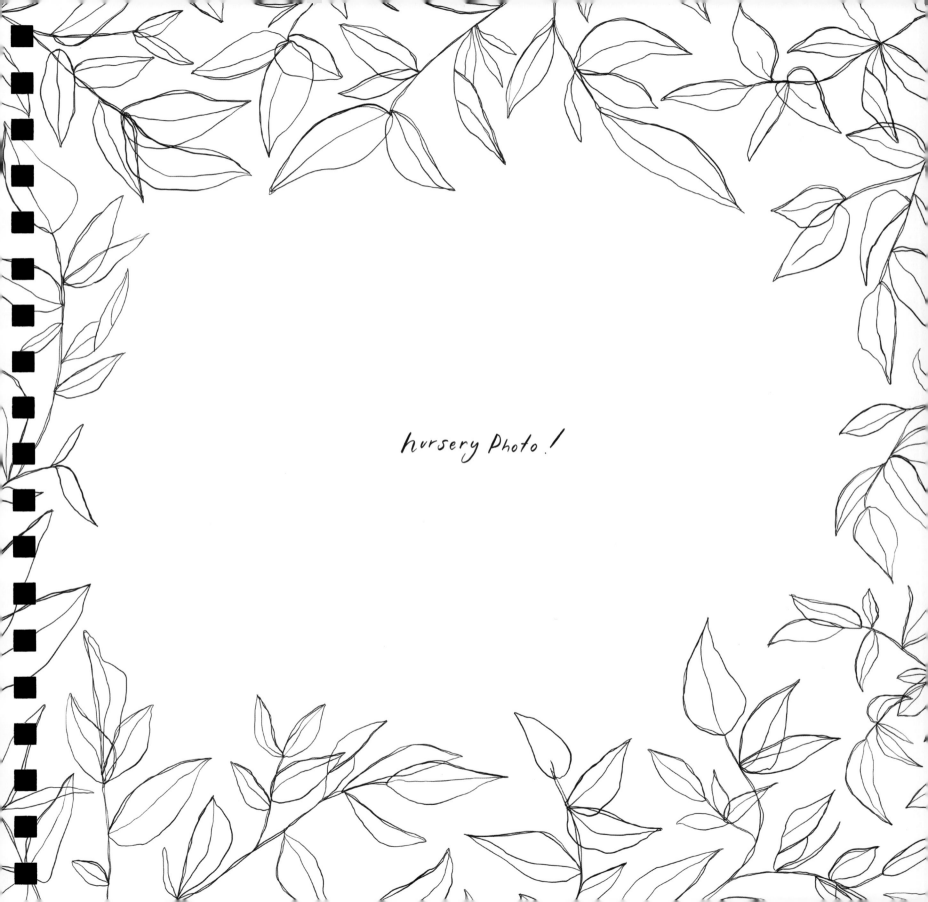

nursery photo!

Name: _____

Date: _____

Message: _____

_____

_____

_____

_____

Name: _____

Date: _____

Message: _____

_____

_____

_____

Messages from 1st Visitors

Messages from 1st Visitors

Name: _____

Date: _____

Message: _____

_____

_____

_____

_____

Name: _____

Date: _____

Message: _____

_____

_____

_____

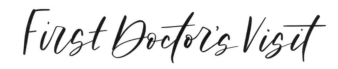

First Doctor's Visit

Doctor: _____

_____

Date: _____

How many days old? _____

_____

Height: _____

_____

Weight: _____

_____

Your reaction to visit: _____

_____

Thoughts: _____

_____

_____

_____

_____

_____

_____

_____

First Real Outing With Baby

Where did you go? _____

_____

How old? _____

_____

Who went? _____

_____

Your reaction to outing: _____

_____

Story about our first outing: _____

_____

_____

_____

_____

_____

_____

_____

Baby's First Bath

Date: _____

Who gave bath? _____

_____

How did it go? _____

_____

_____

_____

_____

_____

_____

_____

_____

_____

_____

First Bath

Add Photo Here!

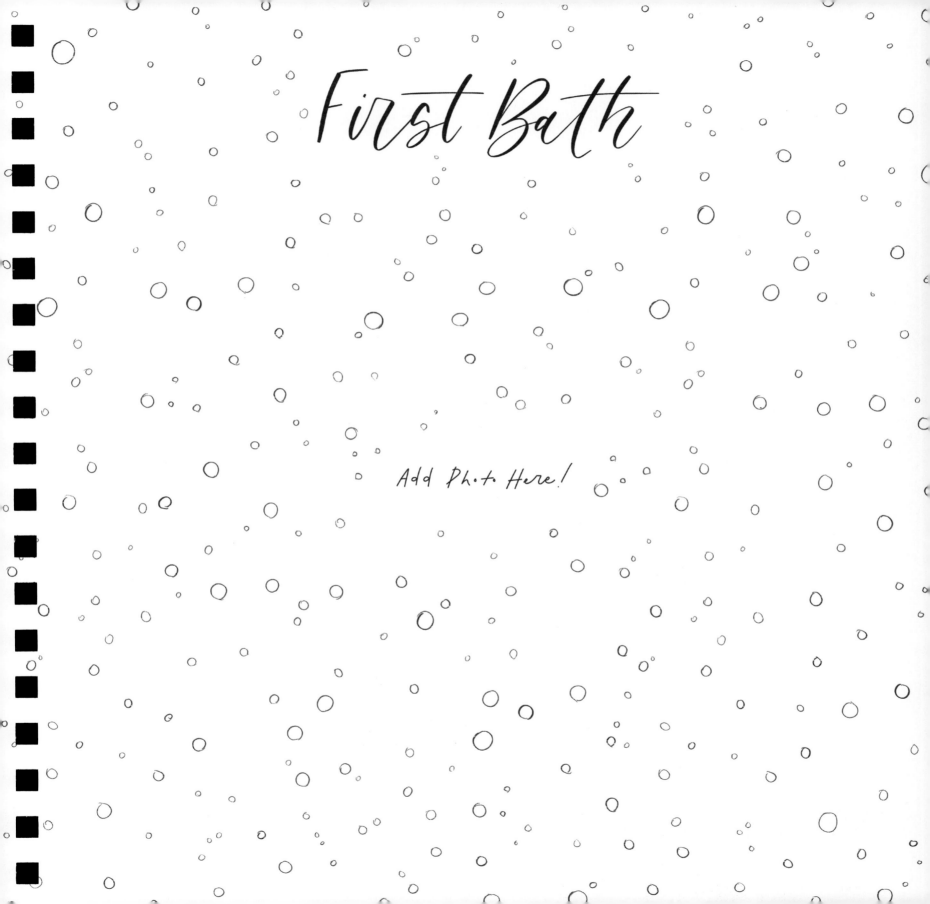

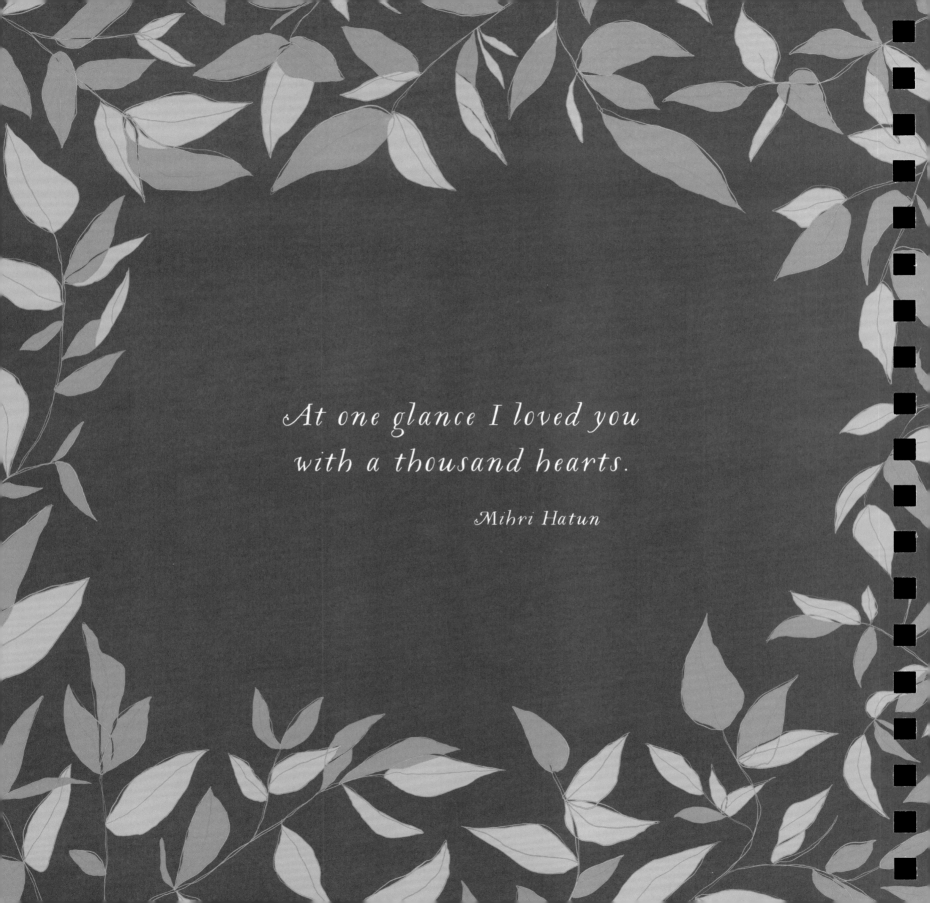

At one glance I loved you
with a thousand hearts.

Mihri Hatun

First Time Apart

Who was left in charge of you? _____

_____

How long were you apart? _____

_____

Where did parent(s) go? _____

_____

Feelings/reactions of both baby and parent(s): _____

_____

_____

Notes from caregiver: _____

_____

_____

_____

_____

_____

_____

_____

_____

Songs We Sing to You

_____

_____

_____

_____

_____

_____

_____

_____

_____

_____

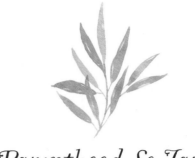

Parenthood So Far

Parenthood described in three words: _____
_____

Biggest challenges: _____
_____
_____
_____

Greatest joys: _____
_____
_____

Surprised by: _____
_____
_____

Thoughts about sleep as a parent: _____
_____
_____
_____

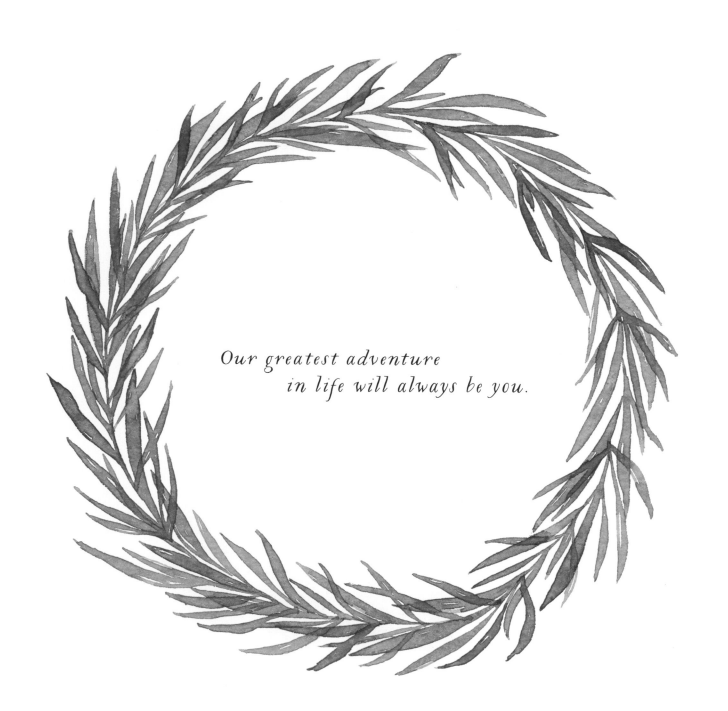

Our greatest adventure
in life will always be you.

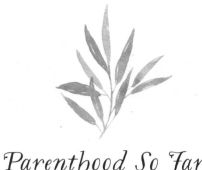

Parenthood So Far

Parenthood described in three words: _____

_____

Biggest challenges: _____

_____

_____

_____

Greatest joys: _____

_____

_____

_____

Surprised by: _____

_____

_____

Thoughts about sleep as a parent: _____

_____

_____

_____

Thoughts about this new life with you: _____

_____

_____

_____

_____

_____

_____

_____

_____

_____

_____

_____

_____

_____

_____

_____

_____

_____

_____

Discovering You

Inside This Pocket

_____

_____

_____

_____

_____

_____

_____

_____

_____

First Year Growth Chart

	Weight/Weight Percentile	Height/Height Percentile	Clothing Size
Month 1			
Month 2			
Month 3			
Month 4			
Month 5			
Month 6			
Month 7			
Month 8			
Month 9			
Month 10			
Month 11			
Month 12			

One Month Old

One Month Photo

Thoughts: _____

_____

_____

_____

_____

_____

_____

_____

One Month Old

Date: _____

Your temperament: _____

_____

Sleep patterns: _____

_____

New developments: _____

_____

Favorite book: _____

_____

Favorite toy (and favorite way to play with it): _____

_____

_____

_____

Likes: _____

_____

Dislikes: _____

_____

Pacifier: ☐   Thumb: ☐   Neither: ☐

Two Months Old

Two Month Photo

Thoughts: _____

_____

_____

_____

_____

_____

_____

_____

Two Months Old

Date: _____

Your temperament: _____

_____

Sleep patterns: _____

_____

New developments: _____

_____

Favorite book: _____

_____

Favorite toy (and favorite way to play with it): _____

_____

_____

_____

Likes: _____

_____

Dislikes: _____

_____

Pacifier: ☐   Thumb: ☐   Neither: ☐

Three Months Old

Three Month Photo

Thoughts: _____

_____

_____

_____

_____

_____

_____

Three Months Old

Date: _____

Your temperament: _____

_____

Sleep patterns: _____

_____

New developments: _____

_____

Favorite book: _____

_____

Favorite toy (and favorite way to play with it): _____

_____

_____

_____

Likes: _____

_____

Dislikes: _____

_____

Pacifier: ☐   Thumb: ☐   Neither: ☐

Four Months Old

Four Month Photo

Thoughts:
_____

_____

_____

_____

_____

_____

_____

_____

Four Months Old

Date: _____

Your temperament: _____
_____

Sleep patterns: _____
_____

New developments: _____
_____

Favorite book: _____
_____

Favorite toy (and favorite way to play with it): _____
_____
_____
_____

Likes: _____
_____

Dislikes: _____
_____

Pacifier: ☐   Thumb: ☐   Neither: ☐

Five Months Old

Five Month Photo

Thoughts: _____

_____

_____

_____

_____

_____

_____

Five Months Old

Date: _____

Your temperament: _____

_____

Sleep patterns: _____

_____

New developments: _____

_____

Favorite book: _____

_____

Favorite toy (and favorite way to play with it): _____

_____

_____

_____

Likes: _____

_____

Dislikes: _____

_____

Pacifier: ☐   Thumb: ☐   Neither: ☐

Six Months Old

Six Month Photo

Thoughts: _____

_____

_____

_____

_____

_____

_____

_____

Six Months Old

Date: _____

Your temperament: _____

_____

Sleep patterns: _____

_____

New developments: _____

_____

Favorite book: _____

_____

Favorite toy (and favorite way to play with it): _____

_____

_____

_____

Likes: _____

_____

Dislikes: _____

_____

Pacifier: ☐   Thumb: ☐   Neither: ☐

Seven Months Old

Seven Month Photo

Thoughts: _____

_____

_____

_____

_____

_____

_____

Seven Months Old

Date: _____

Your temperament: _____

_____

Sleep patterns: _____

_____

New developments: _____

_____

Favorite book: _____

_____

Favorite toy (and favorite way to play with it): _____

_____

_____

_____

Likes: _____

_____

Dislikes: _____

_____

Pacifier: ☐   Thumb: ☐   Neither: ☐

Eight Months Old

Eight Month Photo

Thoughts: _____

_____

_____

_____

_____

_____

_____

_____

Eight Months Old

Date: _____

Your temperament: _____

_____

Sleep patterns: _____

_____

New developments: _____

_____

Favorite book: _____

_____

Favorite toy (and favorite way to play with it): _____

_____

_____

_____

Likes: _____

_____

Dislikes: _____

_____

Pacifier: ☐   Thumb: ☐   Neither: ☐

Nine Months Old

Nine Month Photo

Thoughts: _____

_____

_____

_____

_____

_____

_____

_____

Nine Months Old

Date: _____

Your temperament: _____

_____

Sleep patterns: _____

_____

New developments: _____

_____

Favorite book: _____

_____

Favorite toy (and favorite way to play with it): _____

_____

_____

_____

Likes: _____

_____

Dislikes: _____

_____

Pacifier: ☐   *Thumb:* ☐   *Neither:* ☐

Ten Months Old

Ten Month Photo

Thoughts: _____

_____

_____

_____

_____

_____

_____

_____

Ten Months Old

Date: _____

Your temperament: _____

_____

Sleep patterns: _____

_____

New developments: _____

_____

Favorite book: _____

_____

Favorite toy (and favorite way to play with it): _____

_____

_____

_____

Likes: _____

_____

Dislikes: _____

_____

Pacifier: ☐   Thumb: ☐   Neither: ☐

Eleven Months Old

Eleven Month Photo

Thoughts: _____

_____

_____

_____

_____

_____

_____

Eleven Months Old

Date: _____

Your temperament: _____

_____

Sleep patterns: _____

_____

New developments: _____

_____

Favorite book: _____

_____

Favorite toy (and favorite way to play with it): _____

_____

_____

_____

Likes: _____

_____

Dislikes: _____

_____

Pacifier: ☐   Thumb: ☐   Neither: ☐

Twelve Months Old

Twelve Month Photo

Thoughts: _____

_____

_____

_____

_____

_____

_____

Twelve Months Old

Date: _____

Your temperament: _____

_____

Sleep patterns: _____

_____

New developments: _____

_____

Favorite book: _____

_____

Favorite toy (and favorite way to play with it): _____

_____

_____

_____

Likes: _____

_____

Dislikes: _____

_____

Pacifier: ☐   Thumb: ☐   Neither: ☐

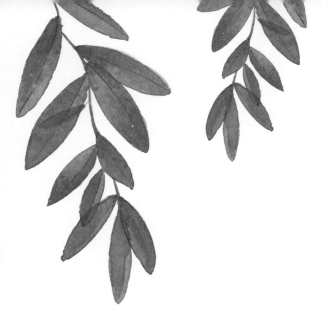

Add Photo Here!

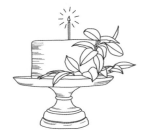

Baby's First Birthday!

How we celebrated: _____

_____

_____

_____

Who celebrated with us: _____

_____

_____

_____

Your reaction to birthday cake: _____

_____

_____

_____

Special memory: _____

_____

_____

_____

Add Photo Here!

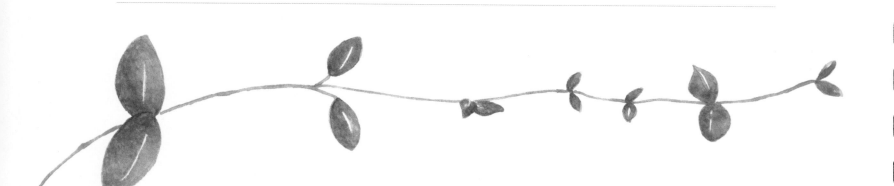

Baby's First Valentine's Day

How we celebrated: _____

_____

_____

_____

Who celebrated with us: _____

_____

_____

_____

Special memory: _____

_____

_____

_____

_____

_____

_____

Add Photo Here!

Baby's First Spring

Things we did: _____

_____

_____

_____

Places we visited: _____

_____

_____

_____

Special memory: _____

_____

_____

_____

_____

_____

_____

_____

_____

Add Photo Here!

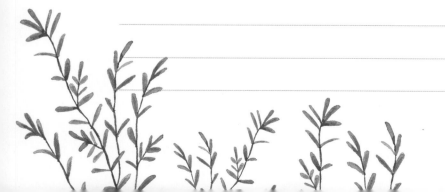

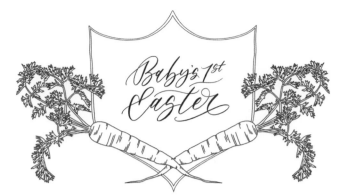

Baby's 1st Easter

How we celebrated: _____

_____

_____

Who celebrated with us: _____

_____

_____

Your Easter outfit: _____

_____

_____

Special memory: _____

_____

_____

_____

_____

Add Photo Here!

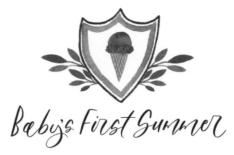

Baby's First Summer

Things we did: _____

_____

_____

_____

Places we visited: _____

_____

_____

_____

Special memory: _____

_____

_____

_____

_____

_____

_____

_____

_____

_____

Add Photo Here!

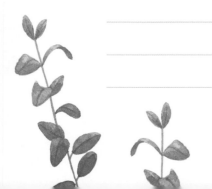

Baby's First Fourth of July

How we celebrated: _____

_____

_____

Who celebrated with us: _____

_____

_____

Your reaction to fireworks: _____

_____

_____

Special memory: _____

_____

_____

_____

_____

Add Photo Here!

Baby's First Fall

Things we did: _____

_____

_____

_____

Places we visited: _____

_____

_____

Special memory: _____

_____

_____

_____

_____

_____

_____

_____

PUMPKIN PATCH

HAYRIDES

CORN MAZE

Add Photo Here!

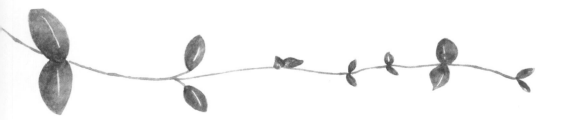

Baby's First Halloween

How we decorated the house: _____

_____

_____

_____

You dressed up as: _____

_____

_____

_____

Where we went trick-or-treating: _____

_____

_____

_____

Special memory: _____

_____

_____

_____

_____

_____

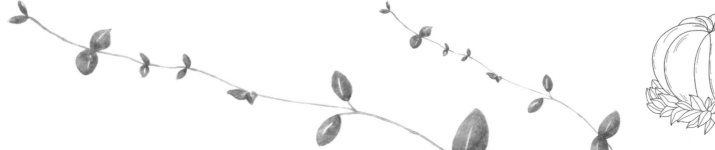

Add Photo Here!

Baby's First Thanksgiving

How we celebrated: _____

_____

_____

_____

Who celebrated with us: _____

_____

_____

_____

What was on our Thanksgiving table: _____

_____

_____

_____

Special memory: _____

_____

_____

_____

_____

Add Photo Here!

Baby's First Winter

Things we did: _____

_____

_____

_____

Places we visited: _____

_____

_____

Special memory: _____

_____

_____

_____

_____

_____

_____

_____

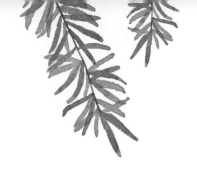

Add Photo Here!

Baby's First Christmas

How we decorated the house: _____
_____
_____
_____

How we celebrated and with whom: _____
_____
_____
_____

A special gift you received: _____
_____
_____
_____

Special memory: _____
_____
_____
_____
_____
_____

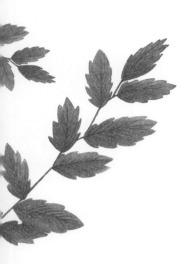

Add Photo Here!

_____

_____

_____

_____

_____

_____

Baby's First Hanukkah

Our Hanukkah traditions: _____
_____
_____
_____

How we celebrated and with whom: _____
_____
_____
_____

A special gift you received: _____
_____
_____
_____

Special memory: _____
_____
_____
_____

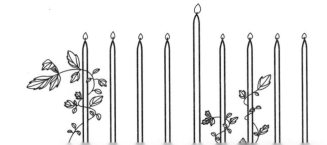

Thoughts after the first year with you: _____

_____

_____

_____

_____

_____

_____

_____

_____

_____

_____

_____

_____

_____

_____

_____

_____

_____

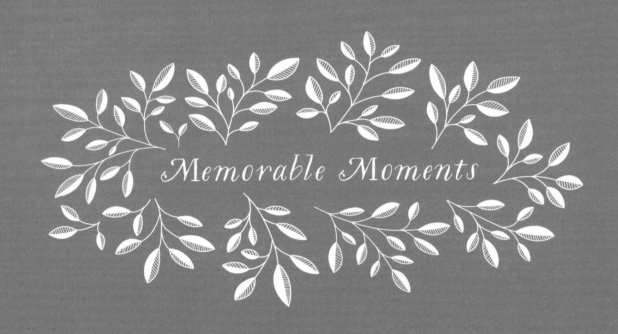

Memorable Moments

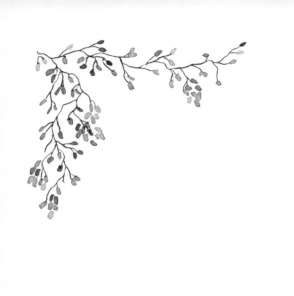
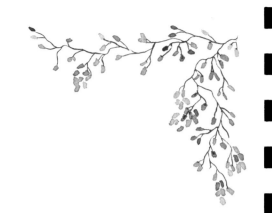
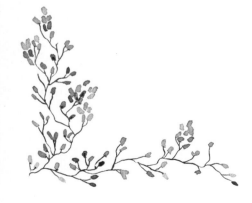
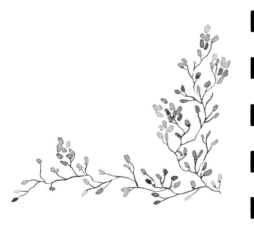

Baby's on the Move

First Time You Rolled Over

Date: _____

_____

Experience: _____

_____

_____

First Time You Sat Up

Date: _____

_____

Experience: _____

_____

_____

First Time You Crawled

Date: _____

_____

Experience: _____

_____

_____

First Time You Walked

Date: _____

_____

Experience: _____

_____

_____

Sleeping Firsts

First night apart: _____

_____

_____

First night in crib: _____

_____

_____

First time to sleep through the night: _____

_____

_____

Description of your special lovey or blanket: _____

_____

_____

_____

_____

_____

First Interactions

First laugh: _____

_____

_____

First babbles: _____

_____

_____

First word: _____

_____

_____

First interaction with technology: _____

    Age: _____

    Device: _____

    Reaction: _____

_____

_____

_____

_____

Things That Make You Cry

First tooth and your reaction to teething: _____
_____
_____

First illness: _____
_____
_____

First boo-boo: _____
_____
_____

First tantrum: _____
    Where? _____
    Cause of the tantrum: _____
_____
_____
_____
_____
_____

Things That Make You Happy

First sweet treat: _____

_____

_____

First trip to the park: _____

_____

_____

First friends: _____

_____

_____

First play date: _____

_____

_____

_____

_____

_____

_____

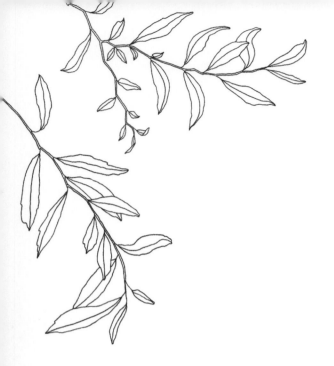

First Haircut

Add Photo Here!

Age: _____

_____

Place of haircut: _____

_____

Reaction: _____

_____

_____

First Tricycle

Add Photo Here!

Age: _____

_____

Reaction: _____

_____

_____

_____

First Adventures in Food

Date	Food	Reaction

Your first ABCs:

Your first signature:

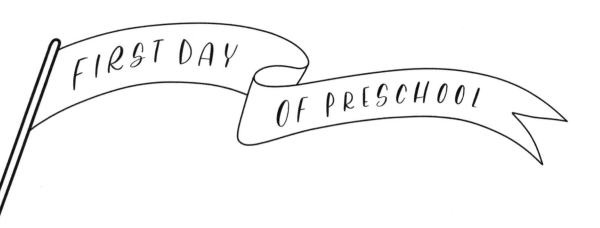

FIRST DAY OF PRESCHOOL

Add Photo Here!

Age: _____

School & teacher(s): _____

Thoughts: _____
_____

First Day of School

Add Photo Here!

Date: _____

_____

School & teacher(s): _____

_____

Thoughts: _____

_____

_____

On watching you experience things for the first time:

Watching You Grow

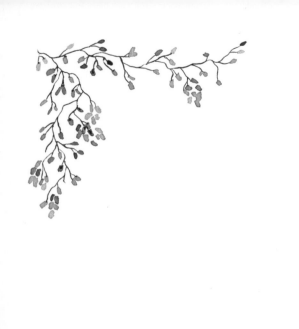
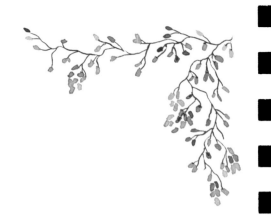
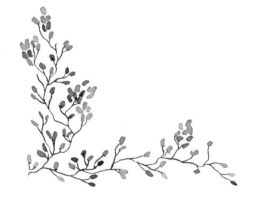
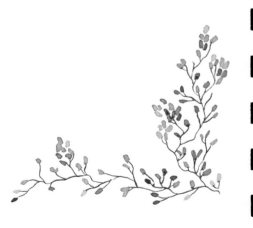

The best thing about memories is making them.

Your Second Birthday

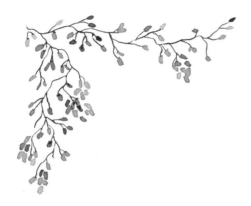

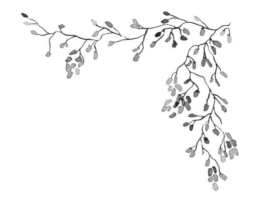

Birthday Photo

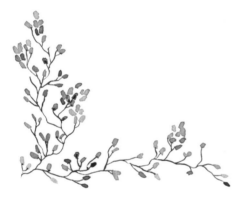

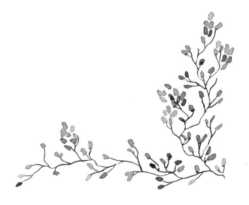

Height/weight on birthday: _____

_____

Who you look like: _____

_____

Your personality: _____

_____

_____

_____

Two-Year-Old Favorites

Favorite movie or TV show: _____

_____

Favorite activity: _____

_____

Favorite toy: _____

_____

Favorite color: _____

_____

Favorite book: _____

_____

Favorite song: _____

_____

Favorite babysitter: _____

_____

Favorite food: _____

_____

Food you dislike: _____

_____

Two Years Old!

Special friends: _____

_____

Places you have traveled: _____

_____

How I love to watch you grow: _____

_____

_____

_____

_____

What you have taught me: _____

_____

_____

_____

_____

My hopes for you: _____

_____

_____

_____

Your artwork at 2 years old:

What do you want to be when you grow up? _____

_____

_____

Your Third Birthday

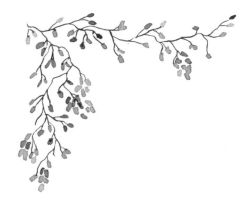
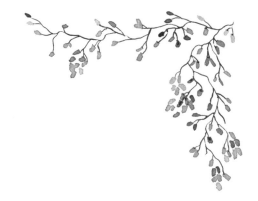

Birthday Photo

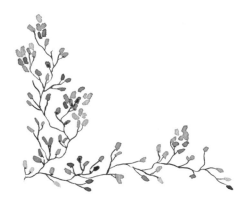
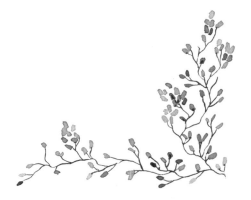

Height/weight on birthday: _____

_____

Who you look like: _____

_____

Your personality: _____

_____

_____

_____

Three-Year-Old Favorites

Favorite movie or TV show: _____

_____

Favorite activity: _____

_____

Favorite toy: _____

_____

Favorite color: _____

_____

Favorite book: _____

_____

Favorite song: _____

_____

Favorite babysitter: _____

_____

Favorite food: _____

_____

Food you dislike: _____

_____

Three Years Old!

Special friends: _____

_____

Places you have traveled: _____

_____

How I love to watch you grow: _____

_____

_____

_____

_____

_____

What you have taught me: _____

_____

_____

_____

_____

My hopes for you: _____

_____

_____

_____

Your artwork at 3 years old:

What do you want to be when you grow up? _____

_____

_____

Your Fourth Birthday

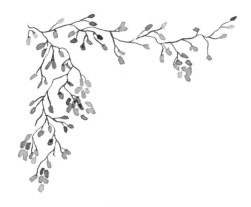 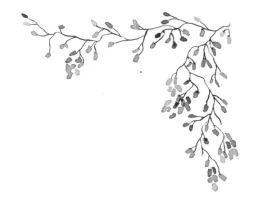

Birthday Photo

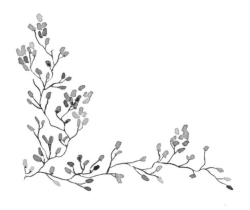 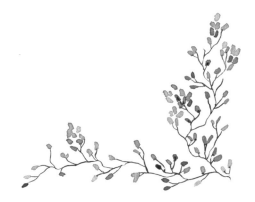

Height/weight on birthday: _____

_____

Who you look like: _____

_____

Your personality: _____

_____

_____

_____

4

Four-Year-Old Favorites

Favorite movie or TV show: _____

_____

Favorite activity: _____

_____

Favorite toy: _____

_____

Favorite color: _____

_____

Favorite book: _____

_____

Favorite song: _____

_____

Favorite babysitter: _____

_____

Favorite food: _____

_____

Food you dislike: _____

_____

Four Years Old!

Special friends: _____

_____

Places you have traveled: _____

_____

How I love to watch you grow: _____

_____

_____

_____

_____

What you have taught me: _____

_____

_____

_____

My hopes for you: _____

_____

_____

Your artwork at 4 years old:

What do you want to be when you grow up? _____

_____

_____

Your Fifth Birthday

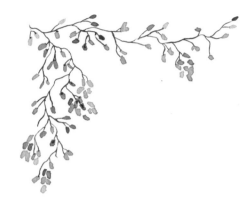
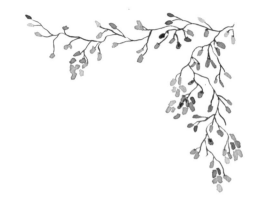

Birthday Photo

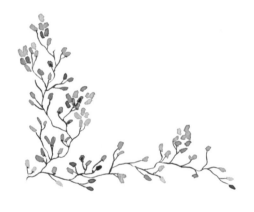
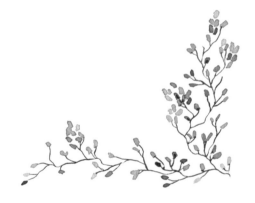

Height/weight on birthday: _____

_____

Who you look like: _____

_____

Your personality: _____

_____

_____

_____

5

Five-Year-Old Favorites

Favorite movie or TV show: _____

_____

Favorite activity: _____

_____

Favorite toy: _____

_____

Favorite color: _____

_____

Favorite book: _____

_____

Favorite song: _____

_____

Favorite babysitter: _____

_____

Favorite food: _____

_____

Food you dislike: _____

_____

Five Years Old!

Special friends: _____

_____

Places you have traveled: _____

_____

How I love to watch you grow: _____

_____

_____

_____

_____

What you have taught me: _____

_____

_____

_____

_____

My hopes for you: _____

_____

_____

_____

Your artwork at 5 years old:

What do you want to be when you grow up? _____

_____

_____

Thoughts for the years beyond toddlerhood:

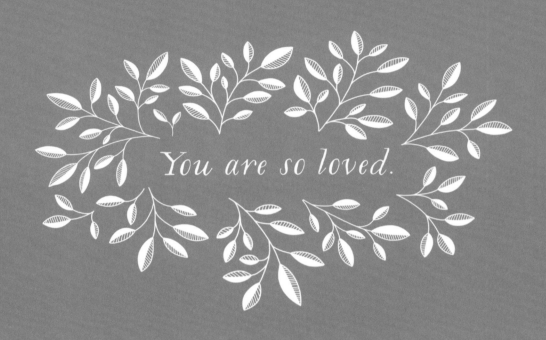

You are so loved.

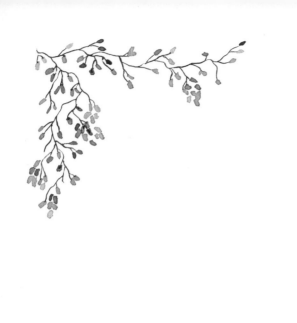
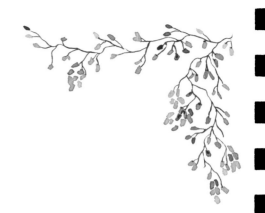
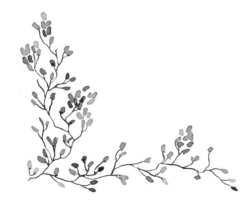
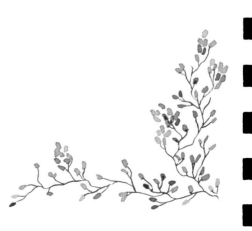

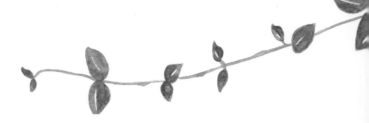

Letters to my Baby

This section of As You Grow is open-ended and completely up to you as to how you want to use it. The brown banner ribbon on the crest of each journal page is intended to house the date you are writing. To get you started, here are a few ideas for how you might use these pages:

People who might want to write in the letter section:

You, the parents!

Baby's siblings

Grandparents

Aunts, uncles, cousins

Close friends of baby

Besides the everyday happenings, a few prompts that baby would cherish from loved ones:

A letter of hopes for baby's future

A letter for high school graduation

A letter for leaving the nest

A letter to future spouse

A letter of advice

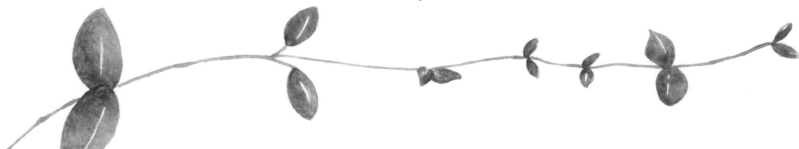

A LETTER
TO MY
BABY

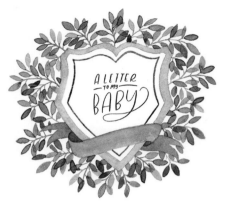

A LETTER
TO MY
BABY

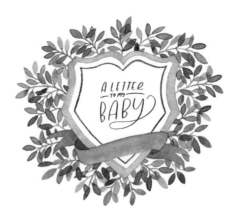

A LETTER
TO MY
BABY

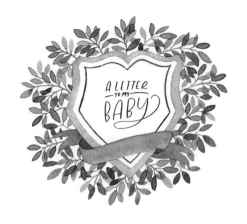

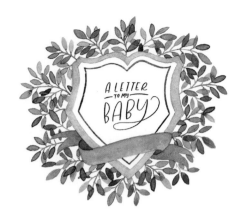

A LETTER
TO MY
BABY

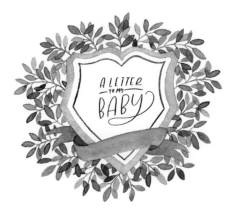

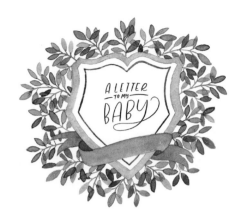

A LETTER TO MY BABY

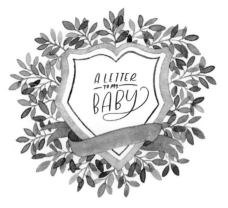

A LETTER
—TO MY—
BABY

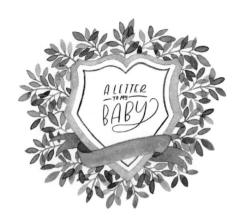

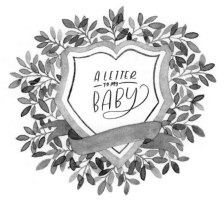

A LETTER
TO MY
BABY

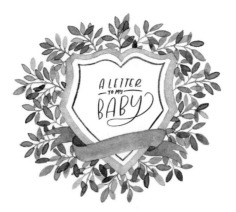

A LETTER
TO MY
BABY

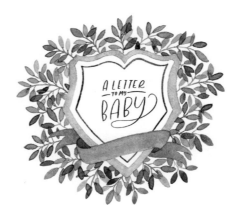

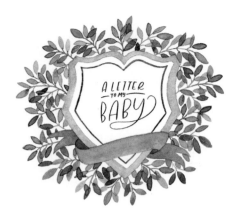

A LETTER
TO MY
BABY

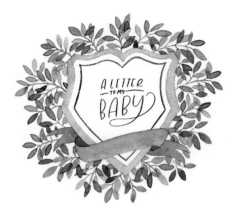

A LETTER
TO MY
BABY

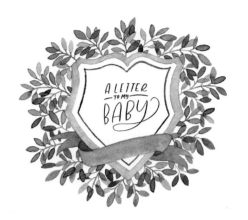

A LETTER
— TO MY —
BABY

A LETTER
TO MY
BABY

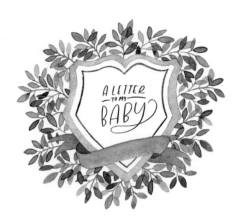

A LETTER
TO MY
BABY

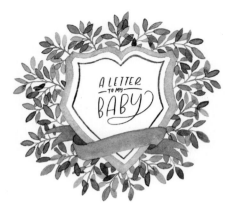

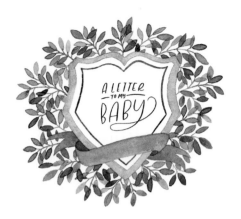

A LETTER
TO MY
BABY

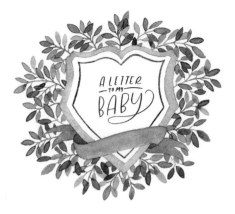

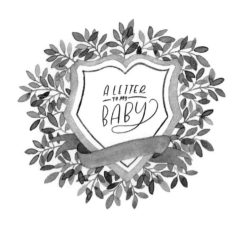

A LETTER
TO MY
BABY

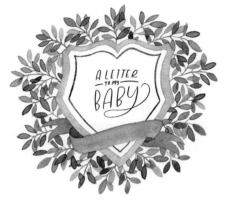

A LETTER
TO MY
BABY

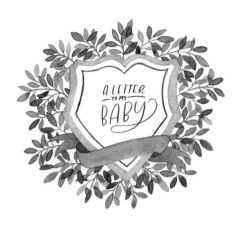

A LETTER
TO MY
BABY

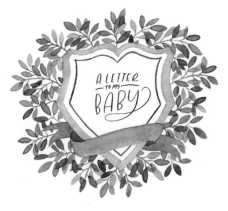

A LETTER
TO MY
BABY

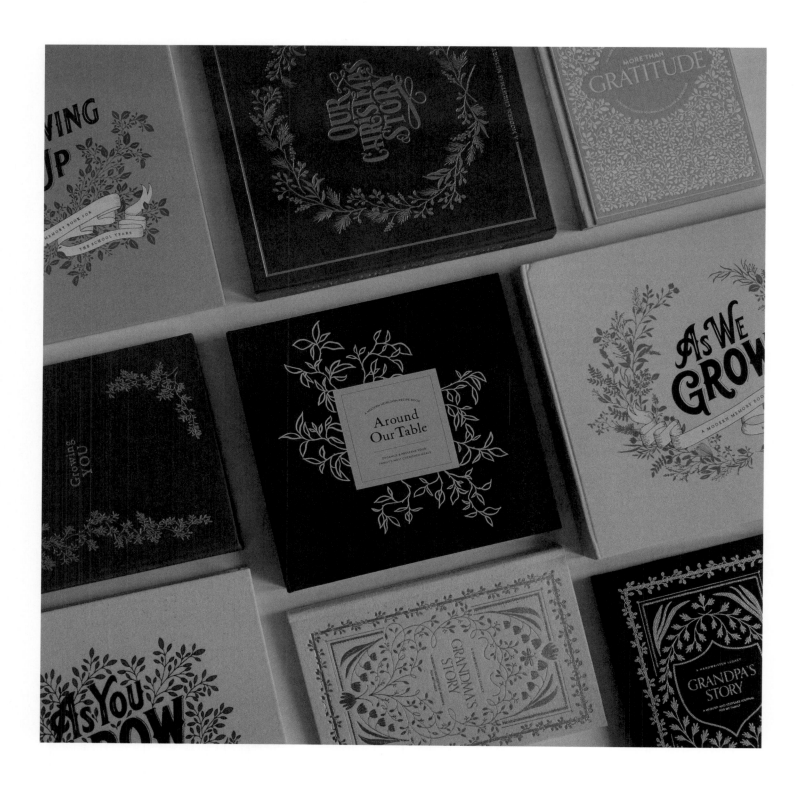

OTHER GIFTABLE BOOKS BY KORIE HEROLD

GROWING YOU : A KEEPSAKE PREGNANCY JOURNAL AND MEMORY BOOK FOR MOM & BABY - *Growing You* is an heirloom-quality book to celebrate and chronicle your pregnancy journey, reflecting on the growth, anticipation, and memories that you want to hold onto as a mother. This journal is the perfect gift for someone early on in their pregnancy.

GROWING UP : A MODERN MEMORY BOOK FOR THE SCHOOL YEARS - *Growing Up* is a modern memory book for the school years and features gender-neutral artwork and space to record precious memories from kindergarten through high school so you can one day pass it down to your grown child.

OUR CHRISTMAS STORY : A MODERN MEMORY BOOK FOR CHRISTMAS - Write down meaningful holiday traditions, record special gifts given or received, save photos with Santa or annual family Christmas cards, preserve treasured family holiday recipes, and so much more! This book makes for a thoughtful gift for a bridal shower, wedding gift, or for a family who loves to celebrate Christmas.

AROUND OUR TABLE : A MODERN HEIRLOOM RECIPE BOOK TO ORGANIZE AND PRESERVE YOUR FAMILY'S MOST CHERISHED MEALS - Preserve all of your favorite recipes, and the memories associated with them, in this heirloom-quality blank recipe book that includes 7 sections to organize your recipes, along with recipe cards, plastic sleeves to preserve new and old recipes, and a pocket folder in the back for additional storage.

AS WE GROW : A MODERN MEMORY BOOK FOR MARRIED COUPLES - *As We Grow* is a place to celebrate and remember the details of your marriage. Record the story of how you live and love and preserve it in writing—a treasure you can pass to your children and grandchildren. It's the perfect gift for the newly engaged couple, the newly married couple, or those who have been married for years!

GRANDMA'S/GRANDPA'S STORY : A MEMORY AND KEEPSAKE JOURNAL FOR MY FAMILY - These two guided journals provide grandparents with thoughtful writing prompts to help them record their most precious moments and pass them down to their grandchildren and families. Beautifully designed keepsake journals, these books are the perfect gift for Mother's/Father's Day, birthdays, or any special occasion.

MORE THAN GRATITUDE - Spend 100 days cultivating deep roots of gratitude through guided journaling, prayer, and scripture. *More Than Gratitude* is ready to meet you where you are, and help you grow in your daily walk with the Lord, through six simple daily prompts. Grab your sisters, neighbors, friends, and family and do this journey together!

YOUR STORIES ARE WORTH TELLING

We believe this in our core, which is why we create the heirloom books that we do. We believe in quality materials, timeless design, and a whole lot of heart. We invite you to visit our website to dive into any of the books in our current lineup and get a deeper look at the contents, purpose of the book, who it's for, and what makes each one special.

WWW.KORIEHEROLD.COM
for more information

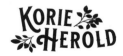

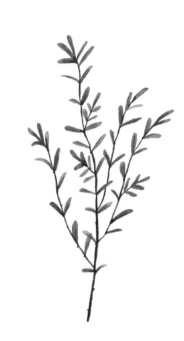

Inside This Pocket

_____

_____

_____

_____

_____

_____

_____

_____